THE
SLEEP
COACH

Also in the Pocket Coach series:

THE CALM COACH

◆

THE CONFIDENCE COACH

◆

THE KINDNESS COACH

A Pocket Coach

THE
SLEEP
COACH

DR SARAH JANE ARNOLD

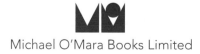

Michael O'Mara Books Limited

First published in Great Britain in 2018 by
Michael O'Mara Books Limited
9 Lion Yard
Tremadoc Road
London SW4 7NQ

A CIP catalogue record for this book is
available from the British Library.

Papers used by Michael O'Mara Books Limited are natural,
recyclable products made from wood grown in sustainable
forests. The manufacturing processes conform to the
environmental regulations of the country of origin.

ISBN: 978-1-78243-917-2 in hardback print format
ISBN: 978-1-78929-016-5 in ebook format

1 2 3 4 5 6 7 8 9 10

www.mombooks.com
Follow us on Twitter @OMaraBooks

Cover design by Ana Bjezancevic
Typeset by Amy Lightfoot

Printed and bound in China

With heartfelt thanks and love,
to my sister, Eva

CONTENTS

'Life is a series of natural
and spontaneous changes.
Don't resist them; that
only creates sorrow.
Let reality be reality.
Let things flow naturally forward.'

LAO TZU

INTRODUCTION

Sleep. What does this word evoke within you? If you're currently experiencing sleep problems, then you might notice that some difficult thoughts and feelings arise. Perhaps there are many things that you do – or have tried – to help yourself sleep better. If these things haven't worked, you may be feeling frustrated, exhausted, isolated, anxious and dejected about your ongoing experience. You are not alone. Insomnia (sleeplessness) affects a large proportion of the global population; sleepless nights can reoccur and worries about this plague many people during their waking hours.

To begin with, this coach will offer some basic information about sleep – what it is, why it happens and how it benefits us. It will then move to introduce the experience of insomnia – what it is, how it's triggered and its impact upon us. From here, if you're willing, we'll embark upon a journey of understanding, acceptance and change that will help you to constructively respond to your personal experience of sleeplessness.

Sleep is a universal, shared experience. It's something that all of us do, and it's something all of us need. It's defined by:

- A period of rest and reduced activity, during which we leave 'waking consciousness', though the brain remains active.

- An archetypal posture of lying down, or sitting up, with the eyes closed.

- A decrease in our responses to external stimuli, such as sounds.

- Changes in brainwave activity, cardiovascular activity (heart rate and blood pressure), breathing rate, body temperature and other biological functions (such as cell repair and digestion).

- Two main types of sleep: rapid eye movement (REM) sleep, which is associated with dreaming; and non-rapid eye movement (N-REM) sleep, which transports us into 'deep sleep'. We typically begin with N-REM sleep; then we tend to alternate between N-REM and REM, recurrently, while we sleep.

- The fact that it tends to be relatively easy to reverse (you can wake someone up).

- The fact that it's repeated at relatively regular intervals, e.g., every night.

During the daytime, our 'drive' (need) for sleep gradually increases. Research suggests that a chemical called **adenosine** builds up in our blood, which causes us to feel tired and drowsy. The longer we stay awake, the more adenosine there is and the greater the need for sleep becomes. When we fall asleep, adenosine gradually breaks down in the body, and the pressure to sleep is released; we wake up after sleeping and the cycle begins again (a process called **sleep–wake homeostasis**).

Sleep and wakefulness are controlled and regulated by the brain. When the areas of the brain that promote sleep are active – and those that promote wakefulness are inhibited – we sleep. When the areas of the brain that promote wakefulness are active – and those that promote sleep are inhibited – we're awake and alert.

Each of us has an internal 'body clock' (the **circadian pacemaker**), located within the brain, which works in accordance with the earth's twenty-four-hour cycle of day (light) and night (dark). It regulates daily neurological and biological activities, and influences our **circadian rhythms** (our sleep-wake cycle). As morning approaches, our body clock responds to the light by producing hormones (cortisol, adrenalin and serotonin) that promote wakefulness. As evening draws in, our body clock responds to the darkness, our waking hormones tend to decrease, and **melatonin** is produced – a hormone that helps us to wind-down, feel lethargic and then sleep.

It's not only daylight and darkness that affect our sleep. There are many internal and external factors which influence the amount and quality of our sleep, including our age, mental and physical health, our work schedule, what we eat and drink, the environment that we're sleeping in, medications we're on, or other substances (like caffeine) that we may be ingesting.

Different people require and prefer different amounts of sleep, at different times, depending upon factors such as their age, lifestyle, genetics and the climate that they're living in. Nevertheless, in spite of individual needs, research suggests that around seven to eight hours of good quality sleep per night is optimal for adults.

Whilst there's still more to be learned about why we sleep, it's agreed that good quality, restorative sleep has these positive effects on our physical and mental health:

- It plays a crucial role in babies and children's brain development.

- It supports the body to rest, conserve energy and recharge.

- It enables the body to restore and rejuvenate itself; research suggests that it has a powerful effect on our immune system, and that cell repair and growth are greatest when we sleep.

- It allows the mind to have some respite from consciousness.

- It helps us to *process* new information, *consolidate* memories and *recall* them.

- It helps us to process unconscious, emotional material when we dream.

- It enables us to learn, problem-solve and perform a variety of tasks (when we're awake).

Sometimes good sleep happens naturally, with minimal conscious thought. Other times sleeplessness consumes us, and we simply can't sleep how we want or need to!

◆ WHAT IS INSOMNIA? ◆

Simply put, insomnia means difficulty sleeping. Most of us will experience insomnia at some time during our lives. This may include finding it hard to fall asleep, and then stay asleep, poor quality sleep (when you wake up feeling tired and don't feel rejuvenated), and/or waking up too early in the morning.

There are different types of insomnia. **Primary insomnia** means that there's no pre-existing problem causing your sleeplessness; it's caused by an interaction between your mind and body alone (hence, it's the 'primary' problem). **Secondary insomnia** means that the underlying cause is another issue, such as depression or chronic pain (hence, insomnia is the 'secondary' problem). If insomnia occurs for three nights or more per week, and for longer than six months, evokes substantial distress and causes social and/ or occupational impairment then it's classified as 'chronic' or severe.

Stress and distress are common features of insomnia. It can be very challenging when you feel the need to sleep; your body is fatigued and yet your mind is frozen in a state of stress (**hyperarousal**), which prevents you from sleeping. Naturally, we react to this situation by struggling with the experience, which paradoxically pushes our readiness to sleep further and further away. Many people report feeling tired and unrested the next day, and feeling sleepy in the daytime is common.

Some of us are more likely to develop insomnia than others. Chronic worry, depression, physical pain, high levels of stress, hyperactivity, having a history of sleep problems in the family, etc., can all make us vulnerable to insomnia. However, these vulnerability factors alone do not cause us to experience insomnia. As touched on earlier, there are various internal and external triggers that can provoke insomnia, such as:

- **Stressors:** challenging thoughts and feelings, such as significant emotional or relationship problems, work dynamics, promotion, financial issues, getting married, moving house, pregnancy and bereavement. Both traumatic and pleasant experiences can evoke stress and hyperarousal, which can negatively affect our sleep.

- **Physical health problems** (diseases and conditions): such as cancer, cystic fibrosis, neurological disorders, hyperthyroidism, hypothyroidism, endometriosis, diabetes, Crohn's disease, arthritis and chronic fatigue syndrome.

- **Psychological difficulties:** such as anxiety disorders, clinical depression and post-traumatic stress disorder.

- **Medications:** including those taken for mental health and physical health problems (such as antidepressants and thyroid medications).

- **Stimulants:** such as caffeine and nicotine (both excess of these substances, and withdrawal from them).

- **Alcohol before bed.** Though it can make you fall asleep, it can negatively affect the quality of your sleep and wake you up in the night.

- **Vigorous exercise in the evenings,** which can stimulate the mind and body – making it harder to sleep.

- **Recreational drugs.**

- **Heavy meals before bed and spicy foods:** both can cause discomfort.

- **Lifestyle:** such as regular long-haul travel, jet lag and shift work – all of which can affect our circadian rhythms.

- **Environmental factors:** such as excessive light, noise and temperature; sleeping in an unfamiliar environment, sleeping alone or with someone else.

- **Hormonal fluctuations:** such as those experienced pre- and post-menstruation, during pregnancy, pre- and post-menopause, and with hormone therapy for transgender people.

- **Ageing:** older adults can experience sleep problems associated with their physical health.

- **Having another sleep disorder** such as Sleep apnea, Restless legs syndrome or Night terrors.

Often, when the trigger is no longer there, our sleep returns to normal with relative ease. However, for some, insomnia can continue long after the stressor that's triggered it has gone. Critically, when insomnia becomes chronic, people can (very understandably) begin to fear sleeplessness and the prospect of trying to sleep itself may become a trigger. Vicious cycles of thoughts, emotions, physical sensations, urges and behaviours fuel sleeplessness and can turn occasional insomnia into a significant, long-standing problem.

Chronic sleep deprivation (not sleeping well for a sustained period of time) can negatively impact our emotions, mood, motivation, perception, judgement, attention, ability to focus, and our capacity to learn and remember things.

When we're sleep deprived, we can be prone to irritability and moodiness; it's much harder to access previously learned information, plan effectively and behave in ways that help us. Our muscles become weaker and fatigued, we can feel nauseous, and the mind becomes increasingly on edge. This is why the brain gets so scared when we can't sleep, because it knows that we need sleep if we're to enjoy optimal physical and mental well-being.

◆ RESPONDING TO ◆ SLEEPLESSNESS

Through the course of this book, you'll find information about good sleep and insomnia, along with concepts and techniques that will help you to sleep well when you can, and to cope better when you can't. Specifically, *The Sleep Coach* will:

- enable you to understand insomnia, how it can evoke your stress reaction, why this happens, how our coping strategies can make it worse, and the costs of battling with insomnia

- offer advice on the lifestyle factors, bedroom

environment, evening time activities and means of winding down that can facilitate good quality sleep

- support you to cope well with sleeplessness in the bedroom, including how to manage your stress reaction to insomnia

- offer advice on what to do if you really can't sleep

- provide tips for the day after a night of insomnia

- summarize the key components of a healthy sleep schedule.

The contents of *The Sleep Coach* are primarily inspired by – and grounded in – Acceptance and Commitment Therapy (ACT) and Mindfulness; it draws upon some Cognitive Behavioural Therapy (CBT) concepts, too. All of these approaches have been empirically proven to be helpful for people with sleep problems. It's my sincere hope that it offers you a fresh and helpful perspective on insomnia, and the ways in which you can help yourself when you just can't sleep.

With warm wishes,

Dr Sarah J. Arnold

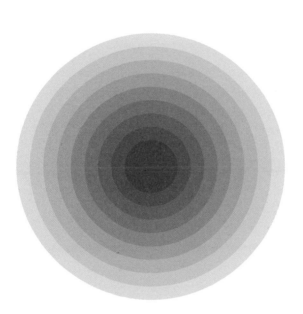

UNDERSTANDING SLEEPLESSNESS

'I know you're tired, but
come, this is the way.'

RUMI

UNDERSTANDING SLEEPLESSNESS

Insomnia and our stress reaction

Insomnia can trigger **stress-related automatic thoughts,** *if* we appraise our inability to sleep as stressful, unpleasant, negative, threatening or unwanted in some way (which we often do). For instance, you might:

- experience lots of expectations in your thoughts, such as 'I should be able to sleep; this shouldn't be so hard'

- predict an unwanted outcome and catastrophize: for instance, your mind might say, 'I won't be able to function tomorrow'; 'I'm never going to get a good night's sleep'

- label yourself as ill – or 'defective' in some way – with fear-based thoughts like 'There's something wrong with me'

- feel helpless and think in 'all or nothing' terms; for instance: 'There's *nothing* I can do to sleep better'.

Have you experienced thoughts like these when you can't sleep? Take some time, and reflect on your thoughts with curiosity. You might find it helpful to make some notes about your observations in a notepad or a diary. These kinds of thoughts are very normal, they tend to reflect the assumptions and beliefs that we've formed about sleep and sleeplessness in our lifetime so far, based upon societal norms and what we've been taught and experienced. For example:

- 'People should be able to make themselves sleep if they try.'

- 'Other people sleep well every night'.

- 'When I can't sleep, it makes me unproductive and incapable the next day'.

- 'Insomnia is abnormal'.

- 'Poor sleep means that there's something really wrong'.

- 'I'm helpless'.

Can you identify any of the beliefs and expectations that *you've* formed about sleep and not sleeping well? Consider their impact upon you. How do they influence what you think and feel; what you do and don't do?

▲▲▲

When we have trouble sleeping, the mind will naturally often try to make sense of it; have opinions and consider if anything can be done about it. When we're stressed, our thoughts tend to be fast-paced, reactive and excessively coloured by fear. This is because the brain is working on the assumption that not sleeping is a dangerous threat that we need to be protected from. It sends us anxiety to try and warn us about this.

If we 'fuse with' (believe and react to) our stress-related thoughts, without noticing what's happening, then they will have a significant impact upon our emotions.

Anxiety, fear, hopelessness, frustration, anger, sadness, panic, disillusionment and feeling overwhelmed are common emotional reactions that are fuelled by stress-related thoughts when we can't sleep. This is because our thoughts and feelings are inextricably linked. For instance, my mind might *think* (*and believe*) 'I can't cope with this!' and I may well *feel* really overwhelmed, anxious and helpless. If my mind were to *think* (*and believe*) that 'I can use this time to rest, and treat myself kindly, even if I can't sleep' – then I'm likely to feel more peaceful, less anxious and more in control.

The brain can't tell the difference between insomnia and a bear approaching you to attack – it perceives each as a threat. Therefore, it sends the same 'Threat! Warning!' signal, which activates the **sympathetic** branch of our **autonomic nervous system** – our **fight/flight/freeze** stress reaction. This defensive reaction is hard-wired into us by evolution, and it's designed to help us keep ourselves safe. When it's activated, we feel it physically – and we're supposed to! Common physical indications of stress are:

- an increase in heart-rate

- breathing harder and faster

- an increase in blood pressure

- stress hormones being released (adrenaline and cortisol)

- an increase in blood sugar (the liver releases glucose for energy)

- muscles tensing

- pupils dilating

- a decrease in digestion processes

- sweating, etc.

Each of these physiological (bodily) reactions serves an adaptive purpose, initially. For instance, our pupils dilate and our vision sharpens so that we can spot the threat; our heart-rate increases, pumping blood to our muscles and oxygenating our blood, so that we can run away *fast* from the threat – or fight it if we need to; stress hormones and glucose give us the energy needed to do this.

Of course, if we're left in a high stress state for a prolonged period, these physical changes can create new challenges. For example, when muscles are taut and tense for long periods of time, we can experience aches and pains, tension headaches and migraines; rapid breathing can trigger hyperventilation and panic attacks.

When 'coping' becomes the problem

It's only natural that we try to reduce the disparity between how things are (sleeplessness) and how we want them to be (restful sleep), because it evokes our stress reaction. In line with what we're hardwired to do (fight/flight/freeze), we'll typically try to **fight** against our sleeplessness with strategies such as:

- trying to force ourselves to relax

- going to bed before we feel sleepy and tired, because we think we 'should' and we believe it will help

- keeping our eyes closed when the mind is awake

- trying to take charge by ordering ourselves to sleep

- bullying ourselves with critical self-talk

- tossing and turning in bed

- trying to argue against – or suppress –
  anxious thoughts with other thoughts

- worrying

- judging our emotions, etc

We try to avoid (take **flight** from) our experience
of sleeplessness with coping strategies such as:

- getting up and doing activities (work,
  checking emails, housework, etc.) for the
  distraction

- taking sleeping pills

- using alcohol or smoking cannabis to avoid
  how we're feeling and provoke sleep, etc

If we've tried to fight off the experience of sleeplessness and we've tried to run away from it, and nothing's worked, we may **freeze** and feel stuck:

- clock-watching or staring at things blankly are common coping reactions.

Unfortunately, reactive (habitual) strategies such as these, that we adopt to try and control sleep, avoid sleeplessness and avoid stress, tend to inadvertently fuel our insomnia and inhibit our ability to enjoy restful sleep. It becomes a vicious cycle.

We experience insomnia and
view it as bad/dangerous

▼

this evokes stress

▼

we worry about the consequences
of our insomnia

▼

37

we try to control when we
sleep, and struggle

▼

we feel more stressed, so we
struggle and react to it more

▼

and our insomnia continues.

We cannot run away from our internal experiences, when we can't sleep and feel stressed, and we cannot control when we sleep; we can only facilitate the conditions (mentally and physically) that will enable us to sleep when we're ready to. If we keep trying – and failing – to control processes that we can't actually control, it will leave us feeling helpless, disillusioned, anxious and overwhelmed.

▲▲▲

The costs of battling insomnia

People, understandably, often go to great lengths to try to protect themselves from experiencing insomnia. Some stop doing the things they enjoy – things that make them who they are – because they become scared that these activities might worsen their insomnia. Others will try lots of different medications in an attempt to 'cure' themselves. Some people will create rigid night-time schedules and rituals, designed to help them sleep.

Of course, all of these coping strategies come with their costs. What's more, even if we do put all of these things in place, sometimes we still won't be able to sleep how we want to. We can spend so much time worrying about our insomnia, thinking about the different things that we can do to make it go away and making alterations to our lives that it can have a huge impact upon our emotional well-being, relationships, social life, physical health and finances. What's more, so much time is spent focusing upon what we don't want (the insomnia) and what we can't change (when we sleep), that we forget to focus on what we *do* want (a rich and fulfilling life!) and what we *can* change (how we respond to sleeplessness).

▲▲▲

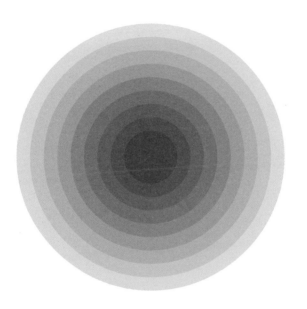

RESPONDING
to
SLEEPLESSNESS

'The beginning is always today.'

MARY WOLLSTONCRAFT

RESPONDING

to

SLEEPLESSNESS

◆ BEFORE SLEEP ◆

In order to prepare for good quality sleep, we need to think about facilitating the conditions that will best enable this; much like selecting the most suitable compost for a particular variety of plant to thrive. This notion is commonly referred to in the literature as 'sleep hygiene'. In essence, it means changing or controlling different aspects of your environment that might interfere with your sleep, and developing helpful habits that will enable you to sleep better naturally.

45

Lifestyle factors

What we consume affects how we sleep. *Caffeine* (found in energy drinks, some fizzy drinks, coffee, teas, chocolate and some painkillers) is a **stimulant** that can keep you awake at night. It activates neurobiological bodily systems that stimulate wakefulness and interfere with the body's natural ability to fall asleep. For instance, caffeine suppresses the effects of adenosine (the chemical I mentioned earlier, which builds up in the blood and makes us feel sleepy). Excessive caffeine can cause unpleasant effects such as restlessness and poor sleep. This doesn't mean that you have to cut out caffeine completely (if you don't want to). However, it's generally recommended to have no more than two to three caffeinated drinks in total per day, and not to drink any approximately six hours before bedtime. A turmeric latte or herbal tea makes a great alternative if you fancy a warm drink later on in the day or in the evening.

Nicotine is another stimulant, found in tobacco products like cigarettes, which can negatively affect the quality of our sleep. Whilst it can be tempting (if you're a smoker) to reach for a cigarette when you can't sleep in the hope that it will calm you, it's important to know that doing so will wake up your body. Nicotine consumption has been linked to disrupted circadian rhythms, fragmented and restless sleep, and sleep being less effective. Try to stop using all tobacco products approximately two hours before you sleep, and avoid smoking if you can't sleep at night.

If you do decide that you want to cut out caffeine and nicotine altogether, then do so very, very gradually. Severe withdrawal from these substances can trigger unpleasant symptoms such as insomnia, anxiety, headaches, intense cravings and increased appetite. It's generally recommended to address insomnia first, restore good sleep – and *then* tackle these addictions.

Alcohol can also negatively affect the quality and quantity of our sleep. Research shows that alcohol, if it's drunk to excess before you go to bed, increases adenosine, which makes you feel tired and fall asleep faster. However, it also increases sleep disturbances in the second half of the night; your adenosine levels lower and contribute to you waking up before you're ready, it can negatively affect your circadian rhythms, disturb REM sleep, cause abnormal dreams and make you get up for the toilet more, too. Many people enjoy a glass of wine or beer with their evening meal. However, if you find yourself drinking more than this on a regular basis in the evening time, then you may want to consider cutting down – both for your sleep, and for your health. When you do drink, try to make your last glass at least four hours before you would like to go to bed.

Do you use these substances (e.g. alcohol or cigarettes)in the evenings before bed? If you do, perhaps you use them to help you relax and feel calmer, combat racing thoughts and promote sleep. Try to understand your intention(s) underpinning your use of these substances, and establish what needs you're trying to meet with your behaviours. Then you can go about replacing some or all of the behaviours with activities that meet the same needs but which benefit you more. For example, you might choose to replace alcohol with meditation practice to promote sleep and meet your need for stress management.

Foods that are high in sugar and those that are difficult to digest can disturb sleep. Eating a big meal before bed is also not recommended. Try to eat lighter meals in the evening, and finish your dinner several hours before bed. If you get hungry later on, choose food that won't disturb your sleep (such as a bowl of cereal with milk). Experts recommend that you consider your fluid intake before bed, too. Avoid drinks that are diuretics (that is, drinks which make you need the loo more than usual). Try to drink enough water, so that you're hydrated – but not too much that it disturbs you. Listen to your body to find the balance that's right for you.

Exercise is another lifestyle factor to be considered. Research tells us that moderate exercise – for at least thirty minutes, three times a week – can help you to fall asleep faster and sleep more soundly. However, timing is everything! Simply put, exercise promotes good quality sleep if it's taken earlier rather than later. This is because exercise stimulates the mind and body, and promotes alertness. If you're experiencing sleep problems, you may find it helpful not to exercise at least five hours before you'd like to sleep.

Bedroom conditions

A *cool* (not cold), *quiet* and *dark* bedroom will help to enable good quality sleep. We sleep best in cooler environments (ideally around 18 °C); as such, some people find it helpful to keep a window ajar during sleep, or use air-conditioning in warmer climates.

Similarly, to address unwanted external noises such as traffic sounds, a snoring partner or noisy neighbours, disposable earplugs can be of great help. Devices like (low noise) dehumidifiers, which emit a soft 'hum', can also aid sleep. It's because this kind of noise is consistent and it drowns out the intermittent, jarring background noises that can jolt you awake or make it harder to fall asleep. What's more, they help to improve the air quality in your bedroom.

As we've already discussed, daylight plays a key role in regulating our sleep–wake cycle. As such, it's been confirmed by science that we sleep best in a dark environment. Some people find it helpful to hang thick curtains (with black-out lining), or wear an eye mask. Remove any other garish light sources, too, such as bright LED clocks, and turn off devices which have 'standby' lights on them.

A good bed with a suitable mattress and pillow play a significant role in your comfort whilst you sleep. Consider the size of your bed, the firmness of your mattress and the feel of your pillow, and make sure that they all suit you. Select inviting bed linen; wear loose fitting, comfortable night-wear made from natural materials (synthetic fibres can cause us to sweat), and have extra blankets ready for when it's cold.

Take some time, when you can, and think about your bedroom environment. Is it dark, relatively cool, quiet and comfortable? Is it somewhere that you want to sleep? If not, what can you do to change this?

In the evening time

There are often things that we need and want to do at home in the evenings. For instance, childcare, preparing food and eating dinner, washing up, cleaning, attending to pets, and so forth. In amongst the 'shoulds' and 'have to's', do what you can to carve out some time for yourself. It's easier said than done, I know, but it's really essential.

In this time, some people find it helpful to pause – and *reflect* upon their day. You might start by asking yourself questions such as:

◄ How have I felt today? ►

◄ What went well? ►

◄ What was challenging? ►

◄ What, if anything, could I do differently next time? ►

Take some time, with a pad or journal, and make some notes about your day. Doing this at the end of each day can help you to express yourself and process your experiences so that your mind can rest more easily. If sleeplessness is a persistent problem for you, then it might be helpful to write about your experience of this, too. Expressing your emotions (in writing, with art or through some other means such as talking to someone) is a very important practice. It enables you to acknowledge what's going on for you in a given moment and then release it (catharsis).

In a similar vein, some people find it helpful to *prepare for the day ahead* before they wind down.

If this is something that you think might be of benefit to you, consider asking yourself the following questions:

◄ What does tomorrow look like? ►

◄ What do I want to accomplish? ►

◄ How will I know when I've done it? ►

◄ How will I accomplish this? ►

Is it essential that I do this
◄ tomorrow, or is it simply desirable? ►
(Prioritize what's essential)

What's my time frame
◄ for this task(s)? ►

A clear picture of tomorrow can enable you to prioritize your tasks, use your time well and feel more ready for the day ahead. Writing a simple, realistic 'to do' list in a diary can help. Once we have a realistic idea of the things that we'll do and how we'll do them, we tend to experience less worry and stress.

During this process, you might notice that some anxieties surface. It's far better, and more conducive for sleep, to *address your worries* and *befriend the anxiety* that you feel, rather than trying to suppress it or run from it. Anxiety is a natural and necessary human emotion. When it's misunderstood, overlooked or intentionally ignored, it can negatively affect our ability to sleep.

▼▼▼

When you notice that you are worrying about something, see if you can first *name* the emotion that you're feeling. For instance, 'I'm feeling anxious'. Then, try to *accept* that this feeling exists for you right now, and remind yourself that you're allowed to feel it. *Validate* your emotion(s) by privately saying to yourself that what you're feeling right now is real and important (even if you don't yet fully understand it). Lean into the feeling, as best you can, and validate your resistance (that feeling of not wanting to). It's not easy feeling anxious! Then, allow your mind to explore it with curiosity, asking yourself:

◄ **'What am I anxious about?' Try to be as specific and realistic as possible, and write it down.** ►

◄ **'If this were to happen, how could I cope with it? What can I do, to help myself and/or the situation?'** ►

Remember, you can't control the feeling of anxiety – or make it go away – but you can respond to it thoughtfully and constructively.

When we greet ourselves with compassion, acknowledge our anxiety without judgement, look at the most realistic 'worst-case scenario' and then plan how we'd cope with it (if it were to arise), our anxiety tends to reduce significantly. If these anxious thoughts come back into your mind at night, then you can gently remind your mind that you have a plan to deal with that particular concern, and you'll attend to it tomorrow.

For more on how to cope well with problems that evoke anxiety and other challenging emotions, check out the additional Helpful Resources on page 123.

Winding down

Sleep isn't something that we can just do; it's something that we *transition into*. We have different types of brainwaves that correspond with how we're feeling and how we interact with the environment around us. **Beta brainwaves** are common in daily life, when we're very alert; problem-solving and decision-making. However, too much time in 'beta' can leave us feeling stressed and drained. **Alpha brainwaves** occur when we engage with an activity that we find deeply relaxing. Research confirms that alpha waves are associated with feeling calm, and they help us to transition into sleep.

When you're ready, you can support your mind to wind down and produce more beneficial alpha waves by doing things that you find nourishing and restful before you go to bed. Gentle pursuits like reading, colouring, meditation and listening to audiobooks about soothing subjects of interest are all great options. Taking a warm bath before bedtime is also an option that's favoured by many. Choose things that absorb and soothe your mind, rather than trying to bore yourself into feeling sleepy.

'Do something boring before bed' is a familiar sleep tip. However, this emphasis on the goal of sleep can actually push our readiness to sleep further away. What's more, it can encourage the mind to wander and leave us feeling unfulfilled. During this time, try to notice your feelings with a welcoming, compassionate and accepting attitude. Don't try and force yourself to relax whilst you're winding down. We can't force ourselves to feel calm and relaxed, any more than we can make ourselves sleep! You might notice some feelings of anxiety and restlessness, for example. Allow these feelings to be with you, and let go of the notion that you're trying to relax. Choose to do something that you find personally meaningful, nourishing and restful instead.

Try to reduce your usage of electronic devices when you're winding down. You may find it beneficial to turn them off at least one to two hours before you decide to go to bed. Research has found that the use of electronic screens (such as those on TVs, laptops, tablets and smartphones) before bed can negatively affect our sleep and sleep patterns. This is because they emit 'blue light' – a type of light that's found naturally in the sun. It stimulates wakefulness, encourages the mind to be active, and suppresses the production of **melatonin** (a hormone and chemical messenger or 'neurotransmitter' that helps us to feel sleepy). Darkness and warm-coloured dim lighting stimulate the production of melatonin, and help the mind and body to relax. Candle light and/or coloured 'mood lights' that glow in shades of orange are best when we're winding down. You can buy remote-controlled colour-changing light bulbs online for affordable prices. (I have several myself!)

Don't go to bed until you feel tired and sleepy

In order to enjoy better quality sleep, we need to address our sleeping pattern and build what's called a healthy *sleep schedule*. If you've adopted some or all of the 'before sleep' habits that we've discussed so far, then you're well on your way to doing this. Waiting until you feel *both* tired and sleepy is key because these are your signals that your mind and body are actually becoming ready for sleep. Many people with insomnia try to force themselves to go to bed at the time that they think they 'should' sleep. Whilst this is understandable (they might have a busy day ahead and really want to sleep), it's yet another example of us trying to force a natural process that we cannot actually control. Remember, we can only enable and prepare ourselves for good sleep. When you feel ready, and you're physically prepared for sleep (that is, you're wearing your sleep attire, and so forth), you can choose to go to your bedroom.

✦ IN THE BEDROOM ✦

When you're in bed, turn off the lights. You are *not trying* to sleep. Remember, you can't force it. You are choosing to lie down in your bed – and rest – because your mind and body have indicated to you (with the tired and sleepy feelings) that you're ready for this.

People who experience insomnia report that this is when they tend to experience an array of stress-related thoughts, challenging emotions, physical sensations and urges. Please know that this is completely normal. Particularly for those of us who've come to associate the prospect of 'trying to sleep' with stress. It's your stress-response in action (the activation of your sympathetic nervous system that we discussed earlier). Mindfulness is great aid for the mind and body in moments like these.

Introducing Mindfulness

Mindfulness is both a *process* (mindfulness meditation) and an *outcome* (which arises from meditation practice; it's sometimes referred to as 'mindful awareness' or a 'mindful attitude'). It's rooted in ancient Buddhist and Hindu schools of thought, religion and spiritual practices. It's also deeply connected with Eastern yogic, Taoist and Sufi philosophies. Humans have been practising mindfulness for many thousands of years, usually as a part of larger traditions such as Buddhism. Since its arrival in the West, mindfulness is now being practised separately from its spiritual, philosophical and historical roots (that is, you don't need to identify as a Buddhist in order to practise mindfulness and benefit from it). Thich Nhat Hanh (credited as the first mindfulness teacher in Europe) and Jon Kabat-Zinn (who pioneered the use of mindfulness in medicine and psychology) are key figures that brought its wisdom to a Western audience, and its popularity has grown exponentially ever since.

To find out more about the fundamental philosophy behind mindfulness, please see the Helpful Resources at the back of this book.

In essence, mindfulness means *tuning in to the present moment – fully and intentionally – with an attitude of kindness, compassion, acceptance, non-judgement, openness and curiosity.* Although mindfulness is an innate human capacity, it is one that requires good teaching, time, practice and patience to develop and master. It's a skill that can be developed formally (via formal meditation practice) and informally (by paying full attention to the present moment with a mindful attitude). It can also be cultivated via practices such as yoga and tai chi.

When engaged in these practices, thoughts are viewed as mental events that recursively come into the mind, stay a while and leave. They are free to flow and come and go, and so are our emotions. Emotions are viewed as non-threatening messengers that can tell us important things about our thoughts, needs and experiences. Physical pain, other sensations and urges are also met with openness and welcomed without reactivity. All of our internal processes are noticed and observed without judgement or control, moment by moment. There is an intention to understand the very nature of the mind, and its connection with the body and our emotions, and our habitual ways of thinking and behaving – and free ourselves from them when they no longer serve us. There is a deep wish to 'simply be'.

Mindfulness teaches us that when we accept the present moment, just as it is, viewing it with a mindful attitude (of kindness, compassion, acceptance, non-judgement, openness and curiosity), and when we accept our suffering, and ourselves, we suffer less. We stop trying to control the things that we can't control (such as the existence of pain), we acknowledge and accept our experiences with gentleness, and we focus on what we can control (how we respond to ourselves and our pain). This is relevant to our battle with insomnia, which is fuelled by us wanting and needing things to be different from how they are.

From this perspective, we can learn how to suffer less with insomnia through learning how to mindfully respond to our stress reactions when we can't sleep. It offers us a new outlook on our suffering and discomfort, and it opens up new and possible ways of managing these things.

There's now a great deal of reliable scientific research evidence that confirms the benefits of mindfulness for our mental and physical health. For instance, when mindfulness is practised for eight weeks or more, it positively affects how emotions are processed and regulated in the brain, thereby reducing psychological distress. It's understood that this may happen because mindfulness promotes metacognitive awareness (our ability to become aware of our own thinking), emotional intelligence, more flexibility (less rigidity) in our way of thinking; it decreases rumination (worry) - bringing us into the present moment instead, it enables us to be less reactive, it enhances our ability to pay attention, and it encourages us to be kinder (less judgemental and more compassionate) towards ourselves and others.

Mindfulness has been found to positively change the brain's physical structure and functioning (a phenomenon called neuroplasticity), helping us to manage fear more effectively. There's also evidence that it reduces **cortisol** (our stress hormone), increases **oxytocin** (the compassion hormone), and improves the functioning of our immune system. When mindfulness is combined with techniques from ACT and CBT for insomnia, it can significantly improve how people sleep, how they think about sleep and sleeplessness, and how they approach these things. Many people report that practising mindfulness, and having it in their metaphorical toolkit, helps them to feel a greater sense of balance, objectivity and mental clarity.

RESPONDING TO OUR STRESS REACTION

In these moments, when we're feeling stressed and overwhelmed by our inability to sleep, we are in the presence of an opportunity. We have the chance to get to know the nature of our mind and befriend ourselves. It's an opening to practise mindfulness and recognize our own suffering with compassion. There isn't 'one way' in which to do this. As such, here are some ideas and ways of being that you can try, adapt and experiment with.

Mindfulness of your internal environment

Your internal environment refers to everything that's within you when you feel stressed or distressed: your automatic thoughts, challenging emotions, physical sensations, pain (if it's present) and urges to do or not do certain things. All of these features are inextricably linked with one another, which can work to our disadvantage (if we're stuck in a vicious cycle) – and to our advantage (if we enable a 'virtuous' or beneficial cycle).

Let's first take a closer look at the presence of stress-related automatic thoughts and urges that arise when we can't sleep (discussed on page 29 of this book), and consider how we can respond to them mindfully.

- First and foremost, *notice* and *name* what your mind is doing by saying to yourself, 'I notice my mind thinking thoughts'.

- Notice how one thought leads to another, to another and another, etc.; observe any emotions the thoughts evoke; note the passing of time when you get drawn into a story (told by your thoughts), and notice when you return back to the present moment; become aware of the spaces in between your thoughts. Observe your mind, without judging it (as best you can).

- If you experience thoughts that express your wish for sleep, such as 'I want to be asleep', validate your wish with compassion. It's normal. Observe other fact-based thoughts, too, like 'My mind feels very awake right now'. Accept that this is simply a part of your reality in this moment. You can't control it, and you don't need to.

- Notice your mind longing for particular things, like sleep, and practise acceptance of these thoughts. They reflect the fact that your mind is struggling with your reality at the moment, and this is completely understandable.

- Allow yourself to be curious about the kinds of things that are coming up for you at this time. If you notice the presence of anxious thoughts, see if you can respect their presence. Your mind isn't trying to hurt you. It might bring to mind other things that are bothering you, too. Pause for a moment, and see if you can appreciate what a wondrous thing your mind is. Using its survival instinct, it's trying to keep you safe from potential threats to your well-being. Noticing what your mind is trying to do, and truly appreciating it, can help you to feel less reactive.

- See if you can consciously *allow* these thoughts to be with you, and try to *accept* their presence. By doing so, you are giving your mind a very powerful message: the fact that you are not struggling with them is telling your brain that they are not a threat. As a result, your stress reaction to them will reduce and your emotions will settle.

It takes time to learn how to be open and non-reactive with difficult thoughts; our primitive instincts tell us to close up and push them away – like a hedgehog curling up into a tight ball, trying to protect itself from a threat. However, if we're to stop ourselves from getting caught in emotional vicious cycles, then we need to drop the struggle with our thoughts and let them be with us. This isn't the same as giving in, and you don't need to like the thoughts. You're simply recognizing a fact: that struggling with them will cause you to suffer more.

There's a technique in ACT called **thought defusion**, which can be of help in these moments. One way of practising this is to use the phrase *'I'm having a thought that ...* [before your raw thought]'. So, for instance, 'I'm having a thought that I'll have a terrible day tomorrow.' If your mind is left to its own devices, it may well latch on to that thought: 'I'll have a terrible day tomorrow'; it will believe it and react to it (a process called **fusion**). It will most likely go on to create a whole stress-related story about why your day will be terrible, what the consequences will be and how this will hurt you. When we notice these kinds of thoughts, and add in front of them 'I'm having a thought that ...'it helps us to 'defuse' from their content. That is, it:

1. helps us to remember that it's just a thought, or a collection of thoughts, which may or may not be true or helpful.

2. supports us to look at the thought from a distance, with more objectivity. As such, we're less likely to get swept away in them.

Another defusion technique, that can be very helpful, is to *name the voice that's talking*. So, for example, you might have a thought: 'I won't be able to function tomorrow.' See if you can pause, in the moment, and see this thought (and those like it) for what they are. It *is the voice of fear*. Your mind is scared, understandably, that your sleeplessness will have a really negative impact upon you. You can reply to your mind by saying, 'that's the voice of fear'. See if you can add in some compassionate self-talk, too, such as, 'There's no wonder you're afraid. It's so hard, feeling this tired yet not being able to sleep'. If there's a grain of truth here, and you really believe that your functioning will be negatively affected, then consider what you can do about this. What are the options? How could you help yourself if this does happen?

When you're suffering with sleeplessness, self-compassion is absolutely essential. It's so easy for stress-related thoughts to take hold. They can be very blaming, critical, judgemental, predictive, catastrophic and over-generalized, and they can evoke a great deal of anxiety. Speak to yourself gently, with compassion. Ask yourself:

'What would I say to someone I love, if they were thinking this?'

and

'What would I like someone to say to me in this situation?'

Try and offer yourself this kindness. You can name the voice that's talking, too, for instance:

'There's my self-critical voice'.

or

'That's the voice of past pain' (the origin of our self-criticism).

74

Notice any urges that you might have to avoid your thoughts, distract yourself from them, or push them away, and name these too. For instance:

'I'm feeling the urge to get up'.

Compassionately respond with words such as:

**'Of course I want to escape
how I'm feeling. It's natural; it's
my flight stress reaction'.**

**'I can try and practise
mindfulness of this instead'.**

See if you can stay in your bed, and notice where you feel the urge in your body. Perhaps your legs, feet and hands feel restless.

Focus your attention on the part of your body where you feel the urge most intensely, and describe the sensations that you're experiencing. For instance:

'I notice warmth in my hands; they're sweating a little and they feel a bit tingly'.

Allow yourself to be curious about these sensations, without judging them. Some people find it helpful to focus on their abdomen or chest as it rises and falls while they breathe. Greet each urge with your attention, and allow it the freedom to be, rise and fall – like the waves of an ocean. Imagine that you're a skilled surfer, surfing these waves. If you get lost in your thoughts, compassionately notice this with kindness, acknowledge where the mind went with a sentence (e.g., 'thinking about...') and then come back to the present moment. We call this technique **'urge surfing'**. There's a link about this in the Helpful Resources section.

▲▲▲

Many people experience the urge to get up and check the time, or simply 'watch the clock', when they can't sleep. This can wake up the mind, reinforce difficult thoughts and create unnecessary stress. Combat this by removing unnecessary clocks from the bedroom and keep your alarm clock or phone out of sight at night. Notice if you get the urge to check the time. Remind yourself that this urge is understandable but unhelpful, and choose not to check the time in favour of your own well-being. You can practise surfing this urge, too, if you want to.

Now, let's reflect upon the challenging emotions that can come up for us when we're unable to sleep. Mindfulness can be very helpful in these instances, too. There are three key skills that we want to practise. They might seem simple, but they take a great deal of time and patience to truly cultivate. These are: **naming** your emotions; **accepting** your emotions; and **validating** your emotions – moment by moment, as they arise.

Different emotions mean and convey different things about our thoughts, needs and experiences. Think of them as messengers. This is why it's very important to be able to differentiate between them, and use language to describe them. To do this, you might say:

> 'I notice that I'm feeling scared'; or, 'I am feeling angry'; or 'I'm feeling sad'.

Let's take each of these emotions in turn and reflect upon its message.

Fear arises whenever we perceive that there's a threat which could harm our life, physical health or emotional well-being (or that of someone we care about). If you're feeling scared, your mind might be concerned about the possible consequences of not sleeping how you want and need to; it indicates that your sympathetic nervous system has been activated, and you're probably feeling stressed. Your mind might need some form of reassurance that – even if you can't sleep – it will not cause you significant harm and you will be able to function tomorrow (even though you might feel really tired). You may need to keep facing the situation that you're scared of, to bring down the fear; and learn about the different things that you can do to give you a sense of control and the belief that you can cope. Look around you and notice that you are safe, even though you're feeling fear. Offer yourself compassion, too. It's so hard to feel like this.

Anger comes up for us when someone or something breaches our boundaries; when a goal or activity, that is essential or desired, is interrupted or prevented; and/or when you, or someone that you care about, is threatened or hurt in some way. Anger, in this context, may well be communicating to you that good sleep, which is essential for your well-being, is being blocked by your wakefulness, and that this disparity – between how things are and how you want them to be – feels really difficult and threatening. It makes sense, doesn't it? Validate this feeling! The anger is just trying to convey its message to you. In response, you might need to take a moment to breathe, and then be kind to yourself. Underneath your anger, there may well be sadness. It's not easy when your basic need for sleep is being prevented; the anger is telling you that this doesn't feel okay.

Sadness usually arrives to tell us about some sort of loss (either real or feared). This might be the loss of someone (bereavement), the loss of something (like our sense of competence), or the loss that arises when things don't work out the way we need, want or expect them to. In response to sadness that's associated with insomnia, and indeed with sadness generally, we need to be gentle with ourselves; increase our experience of pleasant events (such as mindfully engaging with soothing and personally nourishing activities before bed); and do things that help us to feel more in control and competent (like practising the self-help techniques in this book).

It can take time to get used to identifying and **naming** your emotions if you're not used to doing it. Try to use 'feeling words' to describe your emotions, such as *sad, angry, happy, hopeful*, and so forth. 'I feel like I can't do this', for example, is a thought; notice that there's no clear emotion identified here. We can infer that they might be feeling overwhelmed or helpless, but it's not certain. If we are to understand what our emotions are trying to convey to us, then we need to be able to identify and name them accurately.

After we've named our emotions, it's really important to try our best to **accept** their presence. Acceptance doesn't mean liking. We don't need to like the fact that we're feeling stressed or in distress. We're simply acknowledging that these emotions exist, and we're choosing *not* to struggle with them. Remember, our emotions are not the enemy. They facilitate self-awareness, they motivate us, prepare us to take action, enable us to protect ourselves, communicate crucial things to others and evoke others to respond to us. Allow them to flow freely, as best you can, without trying to control them, push them away or hold on to them. Let them be, and observe them as they recursively come and go, intensify and quieten. This is energy that needs to be felt and released; we block it and ourselves, when we try and protect ourselves from it. It's this build-up of unacknowledged, unexpressed emotion that can cause us to suffer more.

Then we move to **validation**. This simply means that you are privately acknowledging that what you are feeling is real and important, and that you're allowed to feel the way that you do. So, for example, when you can't sleep and you begin to feel irritated, you might say something to yourself such as: 'There's no wonder I feel like this.' Even if you don't really understand why you're feeling the way that you are, you're still allowed to feel that way! You're a human being, and all of your feelings are natural reactions to your thoughts and the situation that you're in.

Try not to judge your emotions or call them 'negative'. This will only amplify them and evoke more anxiety. When they're intense, try referring to them as *difficult* emotions or *challenging* emotions. It helps the brain to understand that there's nothing wrong with how you're feeling.

Sometimes, when we get into bed and we want to sleep, we notice uncomfortable physical sensations. For instance, things like tingling or twitching. If we're feeling very stressed about the prospect of not sleeping, then we might notice stress-related physical sensations, such as a racing heart, sweating, and so forth (our fight/flight/freeze stress reaction). The mind, almost instinctively, judges these sensations as 'bad' or 'unwanted', because they feel irritating, unpleasant, threatening or painful, and our resistance kicks in. You might notice thoughts and feelings about your pain, judgements perhaps, and a general sense of wanting it to go away. Resistance is completely natural. However, if we get hooked into this struggle, it can amplify what we're already feeling and make us feel worse.

Being present with unpleasant sensations is an art that mindfulness can teach you, if you'd like to learn. It's not easy, and it takes time, but mindfulness can be of great help when you're experiencing something that you can't change, like an unwanted bodily sensation or pain. Here are some key points to keep in mind, and practise, when you're in bed and sensations or pains arrive:

- First, notice when your mind begins to judge, resist or struggle with your reality, and greet this tendency with compassion. Thank your mind for trying to keep you safe from the things that feel unpleasant, and validate the fact that you began to react in this way; it's completely natural.

- Take a moment to **name**, **accept** and **validate** your feelings (discussed on pages 55–56).

- Now, move your awareness to your body and the sensations that you're currently noticing.

See if you can approach them with curiosity. Try not to judge how you're feeling, and if you do – simply notice this and name it as a 'judgemental thought', and then return the focus of your attention to the part of your body where you feel the sensation(s). See if you can describe them. For instance, 'There's a twitch in my calf; I notice a feeling of butterflies in my tummy', and so on.

- Remember that these sensations are not trying to hurt you, and they will pass – in their own time. Approach them with openness and non-reactive awareness, see if you can allow them to be here with you. With each breath, you're creating space for things to be, just as they are.

- Acceptance is key. Once we accept how we're feeling, then we let go of the fighting: struggling and striving for things to be different from how they are. This reduces our amplified pain.

- Give compassion to yourself for these sensations you are having, and any pain that you feel. Notice if you are suffering and acknowledge this gently. You're doing the best that you can.

- If you're really suffering with physical pain, there are some helpful links for you – referenced on page 123.

Mindfulness can encourage you to develop helpful 'mindful' self-talk – including more realistic beliefs about your experience of insomnia and your ability to cope with it. With time and committed practice, your way of thinking will become less fuelled by stress and fear, and more influenced by acceptance and compassion. This helps to activate the **parasympathetic** branch of our autonomic nervous system more often, which is the system that helps our minds and bodies to feel calm, rest and repair themselves. It also encourages the body to release less cortisol and more oxytocin. Here are some examples of mindful self-talk:

I don't feel ready to sleep yet. That's okay; I can accept this experience without needing to like it.

Many people have trouble sleeping at some point in their lives. I'm not alone in this.

I can have a poor night's sleep and still have a good day tomorrow.

I may feel really tired tomorrow, but I will be able to function.

I can use this time to rest instead, and appreciate being in my bed.

I can practise self-care when I'm
suffering with sleeplessness.

I'm allowed to feel my feelings
about this; it's important to express
them. I can write in my journal.

Mindfulness of your external environment

Many people find it helpful to practise mindfulness
of their external environment, too, whilst they're
in bed. See if you can shift the focus of your
attention, from your internal environment
onto your external environment with a mindful
attitude:

- Tune in to your senses, and really feel
  yourself lying in bed. Find a position that's
  comfortable for you, and see if you can
  really embrace the experience. Notice the
  softness of your duvet, the feeling of your
  head on your pillow, and the warmth of your
  own body. Feel the temperature of your bed

linen; notice the colder spots where your feet and legs haven't been, and the warmth of where they have.

- Use these moments to cultivate your presence, acceptance and non-judgemental attitude. Follow the flow of your breath, and allow yourself to really inhabit the present moment.

- You might not sleep, but you can choose to really rest and be mindful.

- If your eyes don't close naturally, don't force them to shut. Let them be, just like everything else, and rest with your eyes open. They'll close when they're ready to.

- Allow yourself to feel grateful for the safety of your bedroom and the warmth of your resting place, even though you're not ready to sleep just yet.

But what if I really can't sleep?

Psychologists take different perspectives on this. Some say get up (the CBT perspective); others say stay in bed and rest with a mindful attitude (the ACT perspective). If you do get up, embrace your wakefulness once more, engage in a nourishing (soothing) activity, and only go back to bed when you feel sleepy and tired. Alternatively, you can choose to rest and practise the mindfulness strategies that we've discussed in this section; it's really up to you. Feel free to experiment and do what works best for you.

If you do decide to get up – and you are really suffering with your insomnia – then please offer yourself the comfort and care that you need. Compassionate self-care is very important for good quality sleep and emotional well-being, and it's essential when we're in psychological distress. One important act of self-care is to acknowledge *our own* suffering. Insomnia can feel very isolating and distressing. Take your journal or notepad and, in a room with warm-coloured dim lighting, write about your experience now. Write down how you're feeling, what thoughts are there, and about what you're currently finding difficult. Try to offer yourself some kind and reassuring words, like you would say to a loved-one in this situation. Don't strive for peace; it will make it harder to accept your reality as it is right now; it will make you feel more upset and more resistant. Accept your lack of peace, surrender to it, and allow this acceptance to become your peace. Remind yourself of what you *can do* to manage this, both now and tomorrow.

Another important act of self-care is to offer yourself some kind of gentle, compassionate gesture when you are suffering. This gesture isn't designed to make your feelings go away. It's intended to a) acknowledge that you're in pain, and b) improve the present moment that you are in, without making things worse. It's a conscious choice to be kind to yourself, with the belief that you don't deserve to suffer.

What kinds of things help to bring you a sense of comfort, during times of stress and distress? If you don't know just yet, that's okay. It can take time to discover the things that soothe us. Here are some ideas of things that you might like to try:

- Reading a book that's of interest or enjoyment to you.

- Listening to an audiobook. Pema Chödrön's audiobooks are particular favourites of mine; they're incredibly soothing.

- Putting on soft and calming coloured lights.

- Mindfully listening to comforting music.

- Mindfully applying a natural, beautifully scented hand/body lotion.

- Wearing your favourite, comfortable and comforting items of clothing.

- Placing your hand on your chest, and wishing yourself well.

- Using an aromatherapy burner with natural essential oils for relaxation.

- Making yourself a cup of herbal tea (e.g., passiflora, chamomile or lavender).

You might notice some resistance when you think about what you could do for yourself. Doing things differently and reducing your own suffering can feel a little unfamiliar and strange. This is completely normal. Appreciate your mind's hesitation, and do it anyway. You deserve this comfort and care.

If you notice the urge to soothe yourself in counter-productive ways, like binge-eating junk food, drinking alcohol or spending money, then you have another opportunity to practise compassion and mindfulness. You might not be able to control your sleeplessness, but you can choose what you do now. Remember that these escapist ways of managing stress and distress might seem appealing, but they actually deny us so much. They block us from learning how to meet our own needs, they damage our self-worth and foster our reliance on them, stripping away our self-belief that we can cope independently and reducing our confidence. Ultimately, they leave us feeling worse. You have another option now.

◆ THE NEXT DAY ◆

Set your alarm for the same time each day, 7.00 a.m, for example, and get up when it sounds – even if you haven't had much sleep. Do your best to accept that you may feel tired, and commit to your new sleep schedule. Remind yourself why you've chosen to do this. You want to be able to enjoy and benefit from good quality sleep, and you'd like a healthy sleep schedule. Try to remain consistent with your waking-up time, even on the weekends. It will help to 're-set' your body's internal clock.

Resist the urge to nap! Daytime naps can reduce the body's natural drive to sleep at night. See if you can observe the sleepy feelings come and go with mindfulness. Healthy distractions can help, such as going for a walk outside. Use daylight to your advantage too; it will help to keep your mind and body awake and alert, reducing your drive to sleep.

▼▼▼

Values and goals

Another crucial sleep tip, which is often overlooked, is the importance of living a rich and meaningful life (as best you can). The more active and fulfilled we are in daily life, the better our psychological health tends to be and the better we sleep. So take some time now, or when you can, and reflect upon the following questions:

1. If poor sleep wasn't an issue for you, what would you be doing?

2. What makes you happy?

3. What kinds of things would you like to do more of, or start doing?

4. What really matters to you?

5. How would you like to spend your time, whilst you're here on this earth?

6. What kind of person do you want to be?

In order to answer these questions, it's helpful to reflect upon your values. Our values are ongoing principles that matter to us, with which we wish to live in line. Here are some commonly held values:

◆ Friendship ◆

◆ Reliability ◆

◆ Respect ◆

◆ Forgiveness ◆

◆ Fun ◆

◆ Control ◆

◆ Beauty ◆

◆ Friendliness ◆

◆ Authenticity ◆

◆ Bravery ◆

◆ Acceptance ◆

◆ Activity ◆

◆ Freedom ◆

◆ Reciprocity ◆

◆ Adaptability ◆

◆ Patience ◆

◆ Personal growth ◆

◆ Self respect ◆

◆ Adventure ◆

◆ Assertiveness ◆

◆ Community ◆

◆ Connection ◆

◆ Autonomy ◆

◆ Caring ◆

◆ Charity ◆

◆ Determination ◆

◆ Dependability ◆

◆ Contribution ◆

◆ Discipline ◆

◆ Gratitude ◆

◆ Excitement ◆

◆ Fairness ◆

◆ Challenge ◆

◆ Commitment ◆

◆ Fitness ◆

◆ Cooperation ◆

◆ Creativity ◆

◆ Willpower ◆

◆ Wisdom ◆

◆ Self-compassion ◆

◆ Compassion ◆

◆ Curiosity ◆

◆ Generosity ◆

◆ Hard work ◆

◆ Empathy ◆

◆ Encouragement ◆

◆ Honesty ◆

◆ Self-care ◆

◆ Loyalty ◆

◆ Effectiveness ◆

◆ Equality ◆

◆ Love ◆

◆ Order ◆

◆ Openness ◆

◆ Humility ◆

◆ Humour ◆

◆ Intimacy ◆

◆ Justice ◆

◆ Kindness ◆

◆ Sensuality ◆

◆ Romance ◆

◆ Sexuality ◆

◆ Knowledge ◆

◆ Learning ◆

◆ Skillfulness ◆

◆ Supportiveness ◆

◆ Listening ◆

◆ Meaningful work ◆

◆ Mindfulness ◆

◆ Non-judgement ◆

◆ Open-mindedness ◆

◆ Safety ◆

◆ Security ◆

◆ Pleasure ◆

◆ Proactivity ◆

◆ Quiet time ◆

◆ Responsibility ◆

◆ Spirituality ◆

◆ Stability ◆

◆ Trust ◆

◆ Rest and relaxation ◆

▲▲▲

For example, your *goal* (the result you are aiming for) may be to commit to practising this new sleep schedule for the next two weeks. The *values* that underpin this goal for you might be: acceptance; challenge; learning; mindfulness; self-awareness; self-care; and patience.

Notice the difference between goals and values. Goals are concrete things that we aim for, and we either achieve or we don't; situation permitting, we can try again. Our values, by contrast, don't have an end – they're ongoing qualities that we're interested in developing for ourselves. See if you can make a pact with yourself to identify and do some simple value-based things in your waking hours. Maybe make a list of your options. Decide upon one thing that makes you smile, however simple, and do it for yourself today. Start small, and build these new value-based activities into your days and weeks to come.

Gratitude

Gratitude practice (reflecting upon what we're grateful for) is another helpful daytime activity. Every day, in a moment that suits you, see if you can name three things that you feel genuinely grateful for and write them down. For example, 'This morning I feel grateful for my partner's smile; the food that I will eat for dinner tonight; and my ability to hear music.' Consider what your body can do, the people in your life, the privileges that you do have, the things that you are good at, the earth that you live on, etc. If your mind begins thinking about the things that you're currently finding difficult, then acknowledge this with compassion. We can recognize our own struggles and the things that we find difficult on one hand, whilst we also acknowledge what we're grateful for on the other; this helps us to stay in balance.

Gratitude isn't about ignoring what's hard. It's about being able to look at life through a wide-angle lens and see everything that exists, including the good, even when we're struggling. Remember, it's normal for our minds to look past the positives and focus on what's challenging, threatening or difficult. Your mind is trying its best to protect you. You can practise gratitude of this, too!

One final note. Please be aware that your insomnia may return – particularly if you're under excessive stress. This is completely normal, and it doesn't mean that you will go back to square one. Practise mindfulness of the fear-based thoughts that can arise, revisit and use the tools in this book to help you manage your stress reaction mindfully, and treat yourself with the utmost compassion and care. You've managed your sleeplessness before, and you can again.

▲▲▲

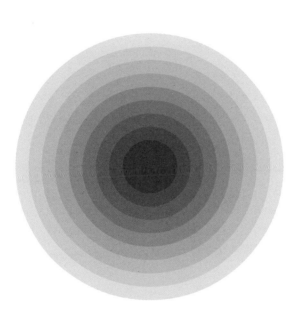

GOOD SLEEP SUMMARY

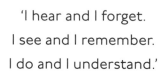

'I hear and I forget.
I see and I remember.
I do and I understand.'

CONFUCIUS

GOOD SLEEP
SUMMARY

Now that we have explored the fundamentals of sleep and insomnia, the stress reaction that can arise from sleeplessness, the science behind this and the ways in which we can learn to cope with it, we have the core 'tools' that we need to enable ourselves to enjoy good-quality sleep.

You can refer back to the previous sections, whenever you need to, to remind yourself of the different tips and techniques that you can use. For your ease - in summary - here, over the next few pages, are the ten key steps needed to help you develop a more healthy sleep schedule and enjoy better sleep:

◆ STEP ONE ◆

Do the things that you want and need
to do in your evening time, whilst
creating some time and space for
yourself – later on – to reflect upon
your day, plan for tomorrow, and
address any outstanding concerns
that you have (as required).

◆ STEP TWO ◆

Embrace your wakefulness and engage
in a gentle, soothing and nourishing
activity before bed (such as meditation,
a warm bath, listening to an audiobook,
etc.) to help your mind and body wind
down. Do this in a calming environment
with orange-coloured, dim light.

Ideally, choose a room that isn't your
bedroom, to help remind your mind

that your bedroom is where you sleep.
If you live and sleep in one room, then
use lighting to change its ambience
– signalling to the brain that there's
a difference between your room in
the daytime and your room at night.

◆ STEP THREE ◆

Don't go to bed until you feel tired and
sleepy (even if it's getting late). This
is very important! These are your cues
that you're becoming ready for sleep.

◆ STEP FOUR ◆

When you're in bed, turn off the
lights. See if you can approach
yourself and your internal world with
a mindful attitude; *name*, *accept*
and *validate* your emotions as they

arise, observe your thoughts, use defusion techniques, and allow sensations and urges to come and go.

Refocus your attention and tune in to your senses; really experience resting in bed. If your eyes don't close naturally, don't force them shut. Let them be, and rest with your eyes open. They'll close when they're ready to.

◆ STEP FIVE ◆

If you find yourself lying in bed for a long time and you're wide awake, and you become very distressed, then you can choose to get up and repeat steps one to three if you want to. Alternatively, you can choose to rest mindfully in your bed. It's your choice; you can experiment with what feels right for you. Compassionate self-care during this time is absolutely essential. Rest as best you can.

◆ STEP SIX ◆

Set your alarm for the same time each day, and *get up when it goes off* – even if you haven't had much sleep. Accept that you may feel tired, offer yourself compassion and commit to your new sleep schedule. Remind yourself why you've chosen to do this. Link it to your values.

◆ STEP SEVEN ◆

NO NAPS. Daytime naps can reduce the body's natural drive to sleep at night. See if you can observe the sleepy feelings come and go,

and resist the urge to nap. Healthy
distractions can help, such as going
for a walk outside. Use daylight
to help stimulate wakefulness.

◆ STEP EIGHT ◆

Remember reconnect with, or establish
your values (what matters to you) and
take steps that will help you to live in
line with these personal principles.

◆ STEP NINE ◆

Practise gratitude on a daily
basis, whilst still acknowledging
what's difficult for you, too. Every
day, in a moment that suits you,
name three things that you feel
genuinely grateful for and write
them down in a personal journal.

◆ STEP TEN ◆

Be aware that your insomnia may
return from time to time; particularly if
you're under a lot of stress. Remember
that this is completely normal. Revisit and use the tools in this book to
help you manage your stress reaction
mindfully, and treat yourself with
the utmost compassion and care.
Remember, sometimes we can't sleep;
it's a normal part of being human.
You can help yourself to manage this
difficult experience, and you can enable
yourself to sleep well again once more.

Try this new routine for two weeks, and see how
you feel!

Insomnia is a challenging experience. Even when
you practise all of the tools and techniques within
this book, it will still feel hard. However, with new

learning, practice, awareness, reflection, trying again and lots of compassion, you can reduce the suffering that you experience when you can't sleep – and you can enable yourself to sleep well when you can. It will take time, require acceptance of discomfort and commitment to your new sleep schedule, but you can do this for yourself. Just take it gently, *step by step*.

▲▲▲

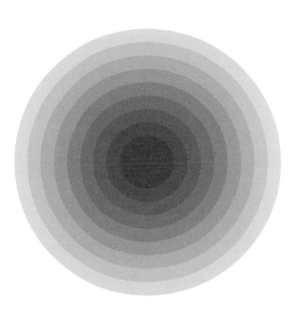

HELPFUL
RESOURCES

HELPFUL RESOURCES

For more information about sleep, and support with sleep problems

www.healthysleep.med.harvard.edu/healthy/

www.howsleepworks.com/hygiene.html

thesleepschool.org

sleepfoundation.org

Arnold, S.J. *The Can't Sleep Colouring Journal.* Michael O'Mara Books, 2016.

Meadows, G. *The Sleep Book: How to Sleep Well Every Night.* Orion, 2014.

Mindfulness resources

www.pemachodronfoundation.org/product-category/books/

themindfulnesssummit.com

franticworld.com/resources

www.tarabrach.com/meditation-radical-acceptance-of-pain/

Arnold, S.J. *The Mindfulness Companion.* Michael O'Mara Books, 2016.

Penman, D. & Burch, V.; *Mindfulness got Health: a practical guide to relieving pain, reducing stress and restoring wellbeing*; Piaktus (2013).

Williams, M.; Teasdale, J.; Segal, Z. and Kabat-Zinn, J: *The Mindful Way Through Depression: Freeing Yourself From Chronic Unhappiness.* The Guilford Press (2007).

Kabet-Zinn, J: *Whereever You Go - There You Are.* Piatkus; New Ed. Edition (2004).

HELPFUL RESOURCES

Addressing emotional difficulties and life stresses can help you to sleep better too

www.thehappinesstrap.com/

www.cci.health.wa.gov.au/resources/
consumers.cfm

self-compassion.org

cedar.exeter.ac.uk/media/universityofexeter/
schoolofpsychology/cedar/documents/Worry_
website_version_colour.pdf

A word of caution

If you are experiencing insomnia or another sleep disorder (like night terrors, sleep-walking, narcolepsy or hypersomnia), and are finding it hard to cope, you may benefit from talking to a mental health professional who specializes in helping people with sleep problems. Seek advice from your doctor or local psychology service to find out about your options.

▼▼▼

ABOUT THE AUTHOR

Dr Sarah Jane Arnold is a Chartered Counselling Psychologist and author. She works in private practice, offering integrative psychological therapy that is tailored to the individual. She supports her clients to understand their pain, break-free from limiting vicious cycles, and respond adaptively to difficult thoughts and challenging feelings so that they can live a full and meaningful life.

Sarah lives in Brighton (UK) with her partner Mine, their dog Oprah, and Priscilla the bearded dragon.

You can find Sarah at:
www.themindfulpsychologist.co.uk
www.instagram.com/themindfulpsychologist

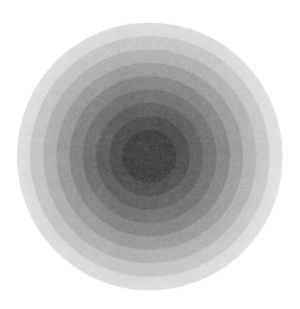